Ayurveda For Beginners

*Balance and Heal Naturally
Using Ayurvedic Principles
and Practices*

Introduction

Do you often suffer from body pains and aches that keep you disturbed at all times? Are you suffering from any kind of bone or joint related pain or discomfort that isn't going away with routine medications? Do you wish to have glowing, soft and supple skin without spending thousands of dollars on laser treatment, expensive creams and skincare products? Do you want to achieve better emotional, physical and psychological health without experiencing any side effects that are likely to affect you if you use medications?

If you answered these questions with a 'yes', it is time you consider trying Ayurveda to achieve balance, harmony and comfort in your emotional and physical health. Ayurveda is an ancient system of natural and holistic healing that is over five thousand years old and originated from the Vedic culture native to India. The discipline was suppressed for a long time, but since the past few decades, it has gained popularity. Various cultures and medicines have their roots in Ayurveda including Traditional Chinese Medicine and Tibetan Medicine, and Ayurveda is now commonly employed in the Western countries and culture as well.

Ayurveda helps to improve your concentration, focus and other cognitive abilities. It also does wonders for your skin, assuages your stress, anxiety and depression, revitalizes your energy and strength, improves your immune system and helps you achieve holistic health balance. You can enjoy all these benefits and a lot more by simply incorporating ayurvedic healing practices into your routine life. If that is what you want, this book is here to guide you in that regard.

Created with the aim to help you become physically and mentally happy and healthy, this book is a comprehensive Ayurveda guide for beginners that helps you heal all your ailments and enjoy a harmonious life through simple and effective ayurvedic healing practices.

Table of Contents

Chapter 1: Understanding Ayurveda

Ayurvedic medicine or commonly referred to as Ayurveda is one of the most ancient holistic healing systems practiced in the world and was created over 3,000 years back. Ayurveda is a Sanskrit term that is translated to 'knowledge or understanding of life' which means that it is a system of practices and techniques that helps you attain greater wisdom about yourself and life in general enabling you to achieve balance in your physical, mental and spiritual health.

Ayurveda emphasizes on complete wellness, which is why all its practices are targeted towards achieving harmony in the external and internal worlds. While its overall aim is to enable you to achieve balance in all spheres of your health, Ayurveda treatments are also geared towards very specific health and emotional problems.

The Principles Governing Ayurveda

We are blessed with five senses, and each of these senses acts as a portal between the external and internal realms through the five major elements in the world namely earth, water, fire, air and ether. In Ayurveda, these five elements are grouped into three preliminary energy types as well as functional principles that are present in everything in the world.

These elements mix and come together in the human body to create three types of energies or life forces known as 'doshas.' The doshas control how the living things work and are of 3 types: vata dosha that is a combination of air and space; kapha dosha which is a mix of earth and water; and pitta dosha which is a unique blend of water and fire.

All of us inherit a blend of these three doshas, but normally one dosha is typically more dominant than others in every person. Every dosha is in charge of regulating and managing a certain bodily function and it is when some sort of imbalance exists in any of the doshas that you start to experience physical ailments, spiritual issues and emotional problems.

Everything in the world has some sort of physical substance, qualities, characteristics and feelings. According to ancient Ayurveda, these qualities referred to as 'gunas' in Sanskrit are classified into 10 pairs of opposites, which makes up a total of 20 qualities such as light vs. heavy.

Basically, everything in this universe has some sort of description and characteristic, and is described using these gunas even the doshas. Ayurveda is based on the foundation of recognizing the surplus or a deficiency of the gunas as this leads to doshic imbalance, which as stated before causes ailments and diseases.

Ayurveda achieves balance by applying the opposite qualities of different things. Leveraging the power of these principles, Ayurveda provides tailor made preventative wellness techniques to cater to the unique needs of every individual.

The 3 Doshas

Let us now dig deeper into the 3 doshas to understand what each entails and governs.

1. Vata Dosha: The practitioners of Ayurveda perceive the vata dosha to be the most powerful of the 3 doshas as it controls the most basic functions in the body such as the division of cells. It is also responsible for your mind related functions, blood flow, breathing pattern, cardiac function as well as the process of elimination of waste through the intestines. There are certain things that create disruption in the vata dosha such as grief, agony, fear, staying up late at night and eating quickly. If you are someone with a dominant vata dosha, you are prone to

developing conditions such as asthma, anxiety, skin problems, rheumatoid arthritis and heart conditions.

2. Pitta Dosha: The pitta dosha regulates your metabolism, digestion process and the connection of hormones with your appetite. Eating spicy or sour foods and spending a long time in the sun are practices that disrupt the pitta dosha. If it is your main force of life, you are susceptible to developing problems such as heart disease, Crohn's disease, infections and hypertension (high blood pressure.)

3. Kapha Dosha: This dosha is in charge of your muscle growth, stability, body strength, immune system and weight. Sleeping too much in the daytime, devouring sweet foods and consuming foods and beverages rich in water or salt are practices that can cause disruption in the kapha dosha. If it is the dominant life force in your body, you are vulnerable to conditions such as asthma, diabetes, nausea, cancer, obesity, and breathing problems.

Ayurvedic treatment procedures are created taking into account your dominant dosha, the problems you are facing and your body type so you get a customized treatment procedure that caters specifically to your problems. Before moving on with that, let us go through the benefits of using Ayurveda in your daily life in the following chapter.

Chapter 2: Why Practice Ayurveda?

'Life (ayu) is a combination (samyoga) of body, senses, mind and reincarnating soul. Ayurveda is the most sacred science of life, beneficial to both humans in this world and the world beyond.'- Charaka

Ayurveda is a system that helps rejuvenate your body, senses, mind and soul so that you feel alive again. Let us get a better insight into its powers and benefits.

Gives You a Deeper Understanding of Yourself and Helps You Practice Self-Love

Ayurveda encourages you to get a deeper and better understanding of yourself by helping you understand the dominant dosha in your system. Once you understand your dosha and its prominent characteristics, you are then able to bring different necessary changes to your diet and lifestyle accordingly. This improves your wellbeing helping you live a better life.

The comprehension of your prominent dosha also enables you to understand the dominant elements in your body and how they affect you. For instance, air tends to show in your mind and body in the form of forgetfulness or boisterousness; fire manifests as anger, digestion and inflammation; and earth is related to your bone and manifests itself in the form of loyalty towards other people and stubbornness. As you become more aware of how the different elements affect you and the dosha you are, you can then find appropriate ayurvedic techniques to achieve optimum balance in your system.

As you take better care of yourself and devote more time to yourself, you start to become more accepting towards yourself. You become aware of your needs and oblige to them, which makes you fall in love with yourself. Self-acceptance and self-love are two incredibly important tools that you must equip yourself with in order to improve the quality of your life.

Helps You Become Healthy through a Nurturing Approach

Ayurveda helps you understand your natural, normal state and how to create a balance in it. You and the environment you live in need to be in harmony with each other to establish equilibrium. Suffering from chronic stress, constant backaches and other issues, physical, mental or emotional are signs and symptoms of imbalance, which you should understand does not happen overnight.

As you become an Ayurveda practitioner, you become more nurturing towards yourself and start to gain better awareness of what brings you discomfort, pain and any ailment so that you can deal with it quickly and achieve balance.

Detoxifies Your Body

According to Ayurveda, there are various types of toxins of which the most commonly occurring one is 'ama' that refers to the waste products of foods and other things such as cells, medicines etc. that builds up in your digestive tract. It is mostly caused by eating too many foods that upset your dosha.

The more there are toxins in your body, the higher your chances of having problems such as inflammation, digestive issues, poor immunity and a higher likelihood of getting cancer.

Ayurveda provides you with relief from these problems by flushing out toxins from your body through different techniques. It also cleanses your body through practices such as yoga and meditation, which further remove toxins from your body helping you achieve peace of body and mind.

Focuses on Preventive Care

Western medicine is mostly focused on treating an existing disease. While this tends to be more of a struggle in trying to put an end to a problem, preventive care actually helps you find relief. Preventive care requires you to take measures beforehand to prevent the onset of a problem and this is one of the most important goals of Ayurveda. You are taught to attune your lifestyle and diet according to your body's unique needs so that you achieve balance in your body, mind and spirit. As you attain this balance, you start to combat diseases and health related problems even before they affect you and improve your overall wellbeing.

Relaxes and Soothes You

Stress is something we experience on a daily basis. Basically, it refers to anything that is perceived as a change, demand or pressure from the environment or from within, and then triggers your stress response, which makes you react/ respond a certain way. This results in different physiological changes including rapid heartbeat and shallow breathing, which increases your stress. While this response fades away in normal circumstances, some people at times are unable to switch that response off once the stressful situation has faded away. They worry so much about a stressful situation that the stress becomes a part of their lives. The stress then interferes with your routine life and everyday tasks keeping you from doing work to the best of your abilities.

Ayurveda offers you relief from these tensions by helping you implement different strategies to combat routine stress according to your dosha and its characteristics. Also, as you release more toxins out of your body, you revitalize your body and mind which promotes overall relaxation in the body.

Combats Early Aging

Many of us suffer from early aging and that manifests itself in different forms including the fine lines and wrinkles on your face and skin. Ayurveda helps you reverse and combat these problems by maintaining balance among your kapha, vata and pitta doshas. This improves your overall health primarily your skin, hair and eyes, which helps you reverse the effects of early and fast aging.

Improves Bone and Joint Health

One of the most notable effects of adopting ayurvedic remedies in your life is improved bone health. Quite a number of people experience joint and bone related issues. Weak bones, pain in joints and conditions such as osteoarthritis are very common nowadays.

Fortunately, Ayurveda can relieve that as well. By helping you bring balance to your vata dosha, which regulates such issues, ayurvedic remedies can easily mitigate your bone and joint related problems, and improve your bone health with time.

Peace of Mind

In addition to improving your physical health, Ayurveda also enables you to achieve peace of mind, clarity and inner contentment. Practices such as meditation and creating balance in your physical being help you think better, rid yourself of stressful situations and enables you to stay calm even in worst case scenarios, focus better on yourself, understand yourself more and pay attention to your needs. This consequently helps resolve anxiety, depression, fears and other emotional disorders providing you with peace of mind.

Moreover, when you shower attention on yourself, you understand your aspirations and goals better, and work harder to achieve them. This along with better self-care in terms of exercising ayurvedic remedies enables you to love yourself more, bringing you a sense of fulfillment. When you feel good about yourself, you find it easier to spread that love and positivity outwards as well and love others, which strengthens your bond with loved ones adding more happiness to your life.

As you have read, Ayurveda is a complete package; it improves each and every aspect of your life and restores balance, peace and happiness to it so you feel better, live better and become better. The following chapters of the book are dedicated to different ayurvedic measures and healing remedies that help you reap these benefits.

Chapter 3: Know Your Dosha Type

The very first thing you need to do to bring Ayurveda into your life and to rightfully benefit from it is to figure out your dosha type. Only when you know what type of dosha is dominant in your system, you can then move on to identifying the most effective and beneficial ayurvedic procedures for your body and mind.

Ayurveda is all about understanding yourself, cleansing off toxic elements from your body and establishing harmony between your body, mind and soul, which can only happen when you are aware of the imbalances in your body, your dominant dosha and your needs so you can then exercise the right measures accordingly.

Let us discuss the 3 dosha types with their characteristics to determine yours:

Vata Dosha

The vata dosha governs all types of movements in your body and mind. It is responsible for maintaining smooth flow of blood in the body, elimination of all types of wastes from the body, flow of thoughts in your mind and your breathing pattern. Your kapha and ptaa doshas are dependent on the vata dosha for all sorts of movements which is why vata is often referred to as the 'leader' of the lot. The following characteristics are dominant in people with an active vata dosha.

1. You have the ability to perform different agility based activities easily. You find it easy to move around, are likely to be quite flexible and enjoy activities involving movement.

2. You walk briskly and enjoy it. Even if you do not like walking a lot, you are a fast walker and do not like to do things slowly.

3. You have a thin and light build. Those with an active vata dosha move a lot and do not rest in one place for long, which is why mostly these people have a lean, slender body.

4. You have light sleep and cannot sleep easily and comfortably at night. This is most probably due to problems with your spleen as it regulates the production of the hormone 'melatonin' that affects the quality of your sleep.

5. You have irregular hunger patterns and are likely to feel extremely hungry at one time, but may starve yourself for

hours at another time. Also, you are likely to have an active eating phase for a few weeks or months followed by one of very less eating.

6. You have a highly active imaginative mind and enjoy thinking about your fantasies, making stories and take interest in activities revolving around creative thinking and imagination.

7. You are likely to be highly enthusiastic and vivacious, bursting with spark and energy and take special interest in things that excite you.

8. While being highly enthusiastic, you are likely to have a high tendency to worry about things and fret to the extent that overthinking takes over your ability to think rationally making you unable to take any action at all.

9. You get exhausted easily even after doing very little work and often complain of pain in your body.

10. You experience frequent mood swings and shifts in mood and may suffer from short temper and anger management problems.

11. You become easily excited and get extremely enthusiastic about things by only thinking about them.

12. You experience bouts of physical and mental energy in bursts that often fade away quickly as well.

13. You are a quick learner as you pick up things and learn information quickly but have a poor memory, and are not able to retain it and recall that same information on time when required.

14. You are likely to experience problems such as flatulence, bloating, brittle bones, asthma, arthritis, and body pains. In addition, you are likely to be more prone to little and big accidents, and stumble or fall a lot in your everyday life. You also have a high likelihood of acquiring Alzheimer's disease.

You need to observe yourself closely for the characteristics and signs discussed above. If you have a highly active vata dosha, you are likely to exhibit at least 7 to 10 of these characteristics. Also, if you have a highly imbalanced vata dosha, you are likely to:

- Have a very dry, rough, thin and scaly skin, which is a problem you often complain about.

- Be underweight and constantly try to improve your physical health and fitness.

- Worry incessantly about your problems, lack of structure and the emptiness you feel in your life and about why you cannot reach the point in life you aspire for.

- Experience racing thoughts often and have a chaotic state of mind most of the time.

- Feel agitated, restless and disturbed constantly.

- Experience and complain about constipation and digestion related issues.

- Not be happy about your lack of stamina and energy, and wish to improve on it.

- Suffer from vaginal issues and dryness often, and are not happy about it.

- Experience extreme discomfort in your joints and even complain about it.

- Experience spells of strange forgetfulness wherein you cannot remember the easiest and simplest of things.

- Be worried about your insomnia that does not let you rest.

If you suffer from or worry about two to four of these issues and experience them constantly for 2 or more weeks, you are likely to have an imbalanced vata dosha. Techniques to stabilize this dosha and the others will be discussed in the following chapters of the book.

Pitta Dosha

Your pitta dosha governs all activities in your body and mind that involve metabolism, heat and any sort of transformation. It is responsible for controlling the way you digest different foods, how you metabolize your sensory perceptions as well as the way you discern between good and bad, right and wrong. Your pitta governs the 'fire' element in your body. The following characteristics are dominant in people with an active pitta dosha:

1. You have a medium build and are moderately strong too, but not too good in tasks involving extreme strength and stamina.

2. It is likely that you have a very sharp thirst and hunger that is not quenched and satiated easily, respectively, and are likely to have a strong digestive system as well.

3. You are prone to irritability and stress, and lose your temper very easily when you are under intense stress.

4. You are likely to have a ruddy or fair skin, which is most likely to be freckled.

5. It is likely you have brownish or reddish hair that is light in texture.

6. You are likely to be extremely sharp, astute and intellectual. You have a knack for reading and a thirst for knowledge, and ensure to use whatever you learn very wisely and tactfully.

7. You are likely to possess an enterprising character and enjoy taking up on challenges in life. While obstacles may scare you at first, they do not dampen your spirits and excite you, and you are likely to embark on different challenges easily too.

8. It is likely that you have articulate speaking skills and are good at conveying your message to those around you very effectively.

9. You are likely to experience problems associated with your pitta including skin rashes, heart problems, acid indigestion, heartburn, liver issues, constipation, peptic or gastric ulcers, diarrhea, nausea, excessive sweating and blood related problems.

Pay close attention to yourself and look for the aforementioned characteristics and signs. If you have a highly active pitta dosha, around 7 to 10 of these characteristics are likely to be a part of your personality. Moreover, if you suffer from imbalances in the pitta dosha, you are likely to fret about the following issues:

- You are extremely critical of people and demand things or people to be a certain way, which can make you a difficult person to be around.

- You often feel intensely angry and frustrated, which makes it difficult to attain peace of mind.

- You are prone to eruptions and rashes on your skin, which worries you a lot.

- You easily become impatient and irritable which often keeps you from doing things properly, thinking rationally and making informed decisions.

- You often wake up in the early hours and then have a hard time going back to sleep.

- You are a perfectionist and are always trying your best to do everything perfectly which oftentimes keeps you from doing anything at all as you tend to wait a lot for the right time to do things.

- You feel extremely hot and become uncomfortable in hot weather, and are prone to hot flashes.

- You suffer from prematurely gray hair or thinning of hair, or both.

- You suffer from loose bowel movement often, which affects your physical health.

- You often complain of indigestion and heartburn which keeps you from sleeping well at night.

If two to five of these concerns worry you a lot and linger on for 2 or more weeks, you have an imbalance of the pitta dosha; hence, you need to focus on restoring that balance.

Kapha Dosha

The kapha dosha governs all the structures related to your body and mind as well as every process involving lubrication. It is in charge of your body weight, lubrication of the lungs and joints, your overall growth and physical development, and the formation of the seven major tissues in your body namely fat, blood, nutritive fluids, reproductive tissues, bones, marrow and muscles. If you have a highly active and dominant kapha dosha, you are likely to exhibit all or most of the following characteristics and features:

1. It is likely you have a very solid and powerful build, and possess great strength. You find it easy to do tasks requiring great muscle power and stamina, and perform well in such chores.

2. You are likely to be quite energetic and are slow, but graceful when in motion.

3. You are likely to be an extremely calm and poised person who maintains his/ her calm in even tensile and stressful situations, and do not get angered very easily.

4. It is likely that you have smooth, pale, oily and thick skin and while your skin quality is good, the oiliness on it disturbs you.

5. You are likely to be a very heavy sleeper and sleep soundly whenever you do.

6. You take your time when learning things and are apparently slow in picking up information, but you are a good retainer and do not forget the information you memorize easily. You recall things passed on to your long-term memory quickly and have a sharp cognition.

7. You have a slow digestion process and do not feel extremely hungry.

8. You are likely to exhibit a tendency towards weight problems and obesity and drive pleasure from eating calorie rich foods. You stuff food on top of your stress and worries, and are likely to be an emotional eater.

9. It is likely you are highly affectionate, forgiving and tolerant towards people. You do not hold grudges and forgive others quickly when they ask for forgiveness. Also, you are likely to have a very loving attitude towards people and spread positivity, happiness and smiles wherever you go.

10. You are likely to take a lot of time when making decisions and then mull over things when you are upset. It takes you a lot of time to get over your pain.

11. You are also likely to be highly possessive about things you deeply care about and have a complacent attitude as well. You are easy to please and satisfy, and tend to change your viewpoints quickly.

12. Moreover, you may suffer from problems such as depression, asthma, diabetes, obesity and cancerous cell growths in your body.

Spend some time closely observing yourself and if you identify 5 to 10 of the character traits discussed above, you are likely to have a dominant kapha dosha. If you have an imbalance in your kapha dosha, you are likely to worry about the following issues.

- Worry about weight management and struggle with weight related issues as you easily gain weight and struggle with losing it.

- Experience lethargy quite often and find it tough to overcome it.

- Complain of sinus problems often that also gets in the way of your physical wellbeing and peace of mind.

- You sleep too much and while you enjoy it, you worry about it because it keeps you from working more and staying active throughout the day.

- Have very oily skin and hair and are worried about them.

- Become overly attached to things, people, ideas, relationships, concepts and life experiences and act obsessively with certain things and people that keeps you from maintaining balance in your life and relationships. Also, your obsessive nature may make it hard for others to feel comfortable around you and enjoy their privacy.

- You do not like damp and cold weather, and in such weather, you may not perform to your optimal level.

- You are likely to be very lazy at times and find it hard to convince and motivate yourself to do something.

- Feel extremely heavy and stiff especially when you wake up, and find that feeling annoying which is why you may not be really active in the mornings.

- Complain of chest congestion often.

If these or even a few of these issues are prevalent in your life, and you often find yourself feeling upset about them, it is because of your imbalance of kapha dosha. There are likely to be certain strong irregularities in your kapha dosha that keep you from living a well-balanced, happy and successful life.

In addition to figuring out your dominant dosha, you also need to understand that all these 3 doshas are a part of you. They are present in each one of us and regulate different functions. You need to pay attention to your dominant dosha and take better care of restoring balance to it in order to feel good about yourself and are able to reach your maximum potential and unlock the finest version of yourself. Apart from that, you need to take care of the remaining two doshas and harmonize them to achieve balance in your life, and are able to manifest a good life.

Now that you are better aware of the 3 doshas and your dominant dosha, you now need to move towards the recovery phase. The following chapters of the book discuss different ayurvedic practices and healing remedies that improve the functioning of your three doshas and help you live your best life.

Chapter 3: Ayurvedic Practices to Balance Your Vata Dosha

Vata dosha has light, dry, cool, subtle, mobile and rough characteristics, which means that to harmonize your vata dosha, you need to work on these qualities and adopt measures and techniques conforming to these characteristics. Here is how you can bring balance and serenity to your unstable vata dosha:

Embrace Small, Slow and Steady Shifts

Before implementing any technique or remedy to stabilize your vata dosha, remember one thing and imbed it in your mind: you need to move in a slow and steady manner, and bring changes in small shifts to slowly adjust to this new routine and very gradually enable your body to settle into the changes you are making.

Successfully adopting a diet and lifestyle habits to balance your vata dosha is not just about following strict dos or don'ts, or being harsh with yourself in terms of the foods you eat, but it is more about paying attention to the overarching patterns and slowly moving your diet and lifestyle towards the right direction.

You need to perceive the entire process like an intention that you are observing to commit yourself to a higher goal; one that would change your life for the better. You also need to see it more like an invitation that helps improve your sense of self-awareness and understanding of the unique needs of your body, mind and spirit.

It is recommended that you start by noticing the different changes you need to make to heal your vata dosha and to gain stability in life. For instance, if you do not sleep properly at night, maybe it is time to cut back on your consumption of caffeine; or if you struggle with maintaining a healthy body weight, maybe you need to adopt better eating habits and increase your intake of whole, nutritious foods and quit the bad habit of eating unhealthy processed foods.

Also, you need to pay attention to how your current lifestyle, eating habits, behavior, attitude and the many other activities you are involved in affect your mind, body and soul. How do you feel about eating certain foods, or when you read fantasy based books, or when you are around certain people?

Focus on what helps you feel calm, positive and good about yourself and avoid things that completely put you off track and make you go through agitation and discomfort of any sort.

As you pay close attention to yourself, your body, your needs and how different things impact and influence you, you slowly increase your sense of awareness and as you develop increased self-awareness, you start to become mindful of yourself and the moment that you live in. This understanding in itself is extremely monumental in helping you choose the right things for yourself and easily distinguish between what's good and bad for you.

This is one thing you need to build the habit of as a heightened sense of awareness helps you bring balance to all the three doshas and not just vata. When you are aware of what things positively and negatively influence you, you can adopt the beneficial ones and slowly nurture habits of those, and avoid the negative influences. With this understanding, you do everything that is required to harmonize your vata, pitta and kapha doshas and improve your lifestyle.

Moreover, it is recommended that you maintain a journal focused on the different changes you bring to your lifestyle to improve it including all the diet changes, routine changes, shifts in sleeping routine and other habits that help you stabilize your three doshas.

When you start a practice, write it down and pay attention to how you feel before and after carrying out the practice. If it improves the way, you have been feeling, stick to it. However, if it does not impact you positively, try something else. Also, give every remedy and practice at least 2 to 3 weeks to show some results because it takes time for your body to let go of a previous routine or habit, adjust to a new one and allow it to influence it.

Observe and draw out a comparison between your body's state and that of your mind before and after working on different practices, and the difference will surely make you stick to the new routine for good. With this understanding, let us now move to the changes you have to bring to your lifestyle.

Prefer Warm Things over Cold Ones

By nature, vata is warm and becomes stable and calm when you increase its temperature and that of your body. By favoring warm things over cold ones, you can create a nurturing, warm and comforting environment for your vata dosha, which slowly restores equilibrium to it. Here are a few things you can try to accomplish that.

- Start by slowly noticing all the foods in your body that have cool energy and lower your body temperature. You need to slowly eliminate these foods from your diet and replace them with those that make you feel warmer. All the frozen foods, carbonated beverages, raw vegetables and fruits, vegetables such as watercress, cabbage, carrots and cucumber, fruits like watermelon and citrus fruits, duck meat and soy products need to slowly go out of your diet. As some of these foods help in stabilizing other doshas such as the fruits, duck meat and vegetables mentioned above, it is best not to completely cut them out from your diet since they are healthy. However, you need to reduce your consumption of these foods and limit them until when you bring back your vata dosha to the equilibrium state. Once you do this, you can slowly return those foods to your diet in moderation. As for the frozen, packaged and carbonated foods and beverages, they need to be slowly reduced and then eliminated from your diet as they actually do you no good.

- Moreover, you need to add more foods with warm energy to your diet. These foods include chilies, onions, ginger, porridge, papaya, banana, beef, fish, pork, eggs, avocado, beets, oats, fennel, asparagus, French bread, pea, rice noodles, jasmine or basmati rice, ramen noodles, almonds, cashew nuts, almond butter, pistachios, sesame seeds, pine nuts, walnuts, pickles, sauerkraut, olives, potatoes, butternut squash, sweet potatoes, corn, mozzarella and butter. Moreover, add spices to your foods such as black pepper, cinnamon, cloves, and mustard, as they too add more warmth to your body and promote stability in your vata dosha. When preparing your meals, use coconut oil, olive oil and ghee more often.

- Often those with an unstable vata dosha have a habit of eating leftovers right from the fridge before warming them. If you do the same, it explains why your vata dosha is deprived of the warmth it needs to function properly. Whenever you eat something, especially leftovers stored in your fridge, warm it up nicely. If you do not like things blazing hot, just warm it to the point that it becomes slightly hotter than room temperature and eat. When warming something, do it on a stove over actual fire instead of using the microwave for the purpose. Natural fire has more energy and warmth, and is not harmful to your body like the rays of a microwave.

- While it is normal and all right to drink cold water on hot days, try to cut back on your intake of cold water. In winters, drink warm water as much as you can and in summers, drink more water at room temperature as compared to cold water.

- Increase your consumption of warm beverages especially in the cold weather. Drink coffee, hot cocoa, eggnog and other warm beverages that make you feel all snugly and comfortable inside. Also, drink herbal teas such as chamomile, tulsi and ginger teas to stabilize your vata dosha.

- If you have a bad habit of skipping breakfast, you need to start taking breakfast. When you wake up, your body is in need of energy and if you deprive it of food at that time, you lower your body's overall temperature, which only harms your vata dosha. Make sure to eat something even if it is a date or two when you wake up followed by some tea or coffee at least 30 to 60 minutes after waking up and then having a nice, home cooked breakfast preferably containing foods that warm you up.

- In addition to eating more warm foods, keep your environment warm and snug too. Add more blankets and throws to your bed, couch and sofas to give them a nice, cozy feel and wrap a blanket around yourself every time you sit or lie down.

- Cover yourself in sufficient layers when going out on a cold day. As for the hot weather, obviously do not wrap yourself up in sweaters and scarves, but do not wear extremely thin clothes and do not keep your shoulders bare. Instead of wearing a sleeveless top or strapless blouse, wear a short-sleeved shirt. Instead of wearing short pants and skirts, wear full-length skirts or at least knee-length. This keeps your vata dosha warm and slowly stabilizes it.

- Make sure your room has a warm, comfortable temperature at all times especially in the chilly winters. Use heaters, blowers or preferably natural fire over logs in a fireplace to keep your place warm and cozy. As for summers, if it is too hot, use air conditioners only when you cannot bear the heat otherwise try to rely more on fans and natural air.

- Take warm baths whenever you can especially in the cold season. Allow yourself to relax in a nice, warm, bubbly bath as the bubbles wash away all your stress, dirt and pain. Take warm showers when you are pressed for time to provide warmth to your vata dosha.

- Light candles and nice incense in your house in the evening to create a loving, warm environment.

If you consistently work on these guidelines, you will soon experience a loving, cozy energy inside you that will steadily warm up your vata dosha and stabilize it as well your mood, temper, behavior and general life alongside.

Opt for Oily and Moist Textures/ Things Over Dry Ones

Vata by nature is dry besides being warm and this dryness is the reason why you experience different ailments, have weak bones and suffer from mood swings. To further harmonize your vata, you need to opt for moist and oily things over dry ones. Here are some things you should try:

- Use more ghee and butter in your diet and use these two items along with coconut and olive oils to prepare your meal. Also, take a tablespoon of ghee, coconut oil or olive oil before going to bed to lubricate your organs and body and eliminate the dryness in your vata dosha.

- Add moist foods to your diet including zucchini, summer squash, yogurt and berries to moisten your body and digestive system.

- Ensure that you eat at least one egg, cooked or boiled while it is warm daily preferably for breakfast to moisten your gut and provide your body with energy throughout the day.

- Slowly cut back on the consumption of dry foods such as crackers, popcorn and white potatoes as they further dry out your vata.

- Do not eat raw vegetables until you have stabilized your vata, which you will know once your health issues start to disappear. Raw vegetables and foods only make your vata drier, which exacerbates your problems.

- When you shower or bathe, allow your body to dry out on its own instead of using a towel every time. If you need to use a towel, gently dab it on your body and use a smooth textured towel instead of one with a rough texture. Leave your body slightly moist and apply a soothing lotion preferably one containing chamomile, lavender or cucumber on your entire body and enjoy the soothing feeling. Massage your body with olive oil at least once a weak to slowly overcome the dryness of your vata dosha.

- Before going to bed, massage petroleum jelly, coconut oil or olive oil on your feet especially your heels and then wear warm socks on your feet. Your heels are connected to your vata dosha so when you provide them with moisture, you lubricate your vata, which restores balance to it.

- Massage your hair and scalp with coconut, almond or mustard oil and keep it on for at least 3 to 4 hours before washing your hair with a mild shampoo rich in almond or mustard oil to promote moisture and smoothness.

Take care of your body at all times and make sure that your skin does not become too dry and scaly in winters by keeping it moisturized it. Also, use a pumice tone when showering to remove dead skin from your elbows, heels, feet and knees very gently to get rid of any dryness and keep your skin supple and smooth. This also softens and lubricates your vata dosha.

Opt for Smooth Things over Rough Ones

This is closely related to the previous ones. Just as you need to take care to keep your vata moist and soft, you need to ensure it does not get in touch with anything rough that makes it even rougher. As vata has a natural characteristic of being rough, you need to favor more smooth textures and things over rough ones to balance out vata's roughness. Here is how you can achieve that.

- For some time, reduce your consumption of rough foods like cauliflower, cabbage, broccoli, beans and dark leafy greens. These foods are rough even when cooked; therefore, for 2 to 6 weeks, limit your intake of these foods. When your vata stabilizes, you can have them again, but in moderation. If you do wish to eat them, ensure that you cook them in ghee or olive oil and add the vata pacifying spices mentioned above.

- Eat less of raw fruits and vegetables for a few weeks.

- Drink beverages with a smooth texture such as milkshakes and yogurt smoothies. Avoid drinking carbonated and fizzy drinks at all times and replace them with fresh juices preferably of the vata pacifying fruits such as bananas, peaches, cherries, grapes, plums, berries and mangoes.

- You can also eat desserts and meals that are smooth in texture such as custards, puddings, very moist and soft cakes and creamy soups.

- Wear clothes with smooth and soft textures and avoid those with a fuzzy and rough texture.

- Use soft blankets, sheets, pillows and bed covers when sleeping.

- Use silk in your clothes as well as the bedding as it is soft and keeps you warm as well.

- Wash your face with milk at least once a day to slowly make your skin soft and supple. This not only softens your skin, but also stabilizes your vata dosha.

Favor Things with Nourishing, Stabilizing and Grounding Qualities

In addition to doing the above, opt for things with nourishing, stabilizing and grounding qualities as things, foods and fabrics that are dense and promote heaviness negatively impact your vata. Here are a few practices that can help nourish and ground your vata;

- When eating a meal, do not consume too much in one go. Instead of having large portions, eat meals in smaller portions and have them every 2 to 3 hours so this way, you eat 5 to 6 small to medium sized portioned meals instead of 2 to 4 heavy ones.

- Avoid eating fried foods as they are saturated in oil and promote heaviness. If you have to fry something, opt for shallow frying over deep frying. It is recommended to brush olive oil on the pan or on the food item, you wish to cook/ fry and cook it over light heat. This keeps you light and does not burden your digestive tract as well. Also, it helps stabilize your cholesterol levels.

- Avoid consuming canned foods as much as possible and go for cooked grains, root veggies, stewed veggies and fruits and spiced milk. A lovely type of spiced milk is turmeric milk. To prepare a single serving, take one glass of milk and heat it over light heat and when it gets warm, add 1 tablespoon of organic turmeric powder in it. You can add grounded brown sugar in it too if you prefer sweetened milk otherwise it is best to consume it without any sugar. Mix well, turn off the heat, and drink it when it cools down a little. Consuming this at least once a day is extremely beneficial for you especially in winters. It improves bone health, speeds up the healing of internal and external wounds and boosts your immunity.

- Reduce your consumption of nicotine and caffeine as much as possible. Keep your coffee/tea consumption to around 1 medium sized cup a day. If you smoke cigarettes, try to quit the bad habit. An effective way to do so is to build incremental goals around this commitment. If you smoke 10 cigarettes a day, commit to smoking only 5 a day for week 1. Once you achieve that you can then move to smoking 4 a day for week 2; then slowly 3 a day for week 3 and so on until you smoke only 1 cigarette a day and then gradually make smoking an occasional endeavor and in about 3 to 4 months try to get rid of this bad habit completely. Take as much time as you want to quit this habit depending on your pace and nature, but put in your best effort to do it for good as it will only restore balance into your body, mind and life.

Since the foods you consume play a monumental role in building your energy and influencing your dosha, here are a few more food related do's and don'ts that you should keep in mind to keep your vata happy.

Food Related Do's to Harmonize Your Vata

- Favor more foods that are naturally sweet such as milk, fresh and organic yogurt, nuts, oils, lean meats, ghee, root veggies, rice and eggs. Sweetness is the foundation of a vata balancing diet; hence, by eating sweet foods, you only help your vata grow.

- Also, add sour foods to your diet as sourness compliments other flavors and enlivens them. In addition, it improves your digestion, moistens other different foods, awakens your senses and mind and boosts your energy. All of this helps resolve the health and emotional problems mostly experienced by those with a dominant vata dosha. You can add vinegar, lemon/ lime juice, kimchi, pickle, sauerkraut or sour cream to your meals and salads to spice them a bit and benefit from their sourness. Moreover, fruits like grapefruit, pineapple, oranges and green grapes in moderation are beneficial for your vata too.

- You also need to add some salt to your foods as the saltiness in foods stimulates digestion and appetite, supports elimination of toxins from the body, enhances the flavors of foods and helps foods retain their moisture, which lubricates your vata. When cooking a meal, ensure to add salt per taste to it, but do not overdo it as too much sodium hampers your hearing abilities and negatively affects digestion.

Don'ts Related to Food Consumption

- Avoid eating extremely spicy and pungent foods. While you should add spices to your foods and consume spicy foods to stabilize your vata, have spices in moderation and avoid eating raw turnips, onions, radishes and chilies. Pungent taste increases the roughness and dryness of vata and only worsens your problems.

- Avoid eating bitter food items such as dark chocolate and kale as bitterness is rough and dry and aggravates your vata. You can eat these foods once your vata is balanced.

In addition to working on your diet, also incorporate the following ayurvedic healing remedies to improve your vata.

Yoga Poses to Harmonize the Vata Dosha

Vata contains a mixture of ether and air elements, and is associated with the fall season as well. Yoga poses that focus on grounding your body and calming the air and ether energy inside you work well in stabilizing your aggravated vata.

In addition, yoga is an important component of Ayurveda as it helps sync your body, mind and soul so that you function as one single unit and achieve balance in all spheres of your existence and life. Hence, by doing yoga daily in your life, you

49

improve self-awareness and align all your energies that promotes healing, harmony and positivity in your system.

Here are some lovely yoga poses to balance your ether and space energies and enhance your physical fitness.

Downward Facing Dog

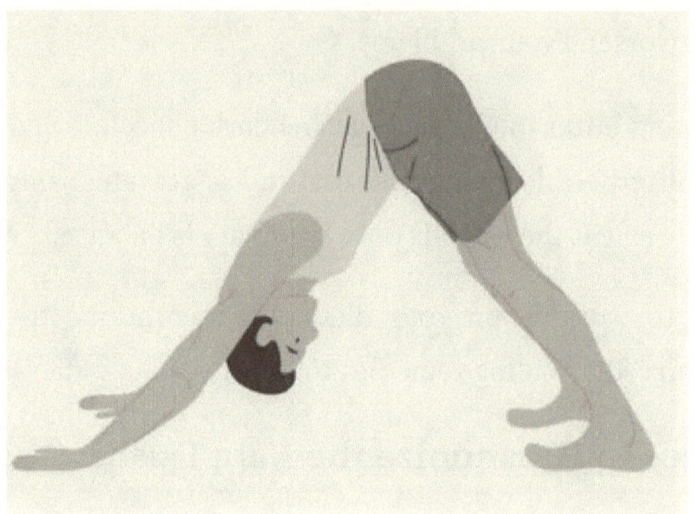

This pose improves the blood circulation in your body especially your head and brain, increases your overall flexibility, strengthens your abdomen, leg and arm muscles, regulates your core and helps you become grounded.

To practice it, stand straight with feet at hip distance apart. Gently, lower yourself down by extending your arms forward and spreading your legs backward to form an inverted V shape. Put your hands on the ground and stretch them while you stretch your legs at the back. Maintain this pose for 20 seconds to 5 minutes.

Mountain Pose

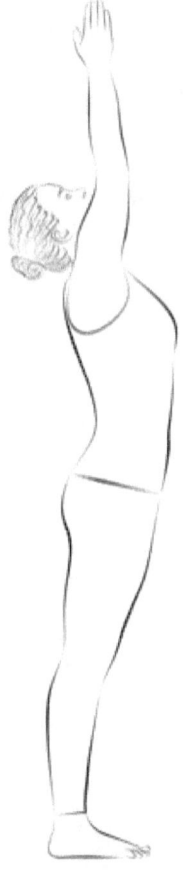

This is a great pose to improve your overall body posture, strengthen your ankles, knees and thighs, improve your self-awareness, boost your power and stamina, firm up your buttocks and abdomen, provide relief from sciatica and steady your breathing pattern.

To practice it, stand straight and keep your feet parallel to one another, heels slightly apart and your middle toes should point forward. Very softly, pull your spine up and open your shoulders and chest while keeping your chin completely parallel to the floor. You can keep your arms and hands raised or bring them down in Namaste pose.

Warrior II

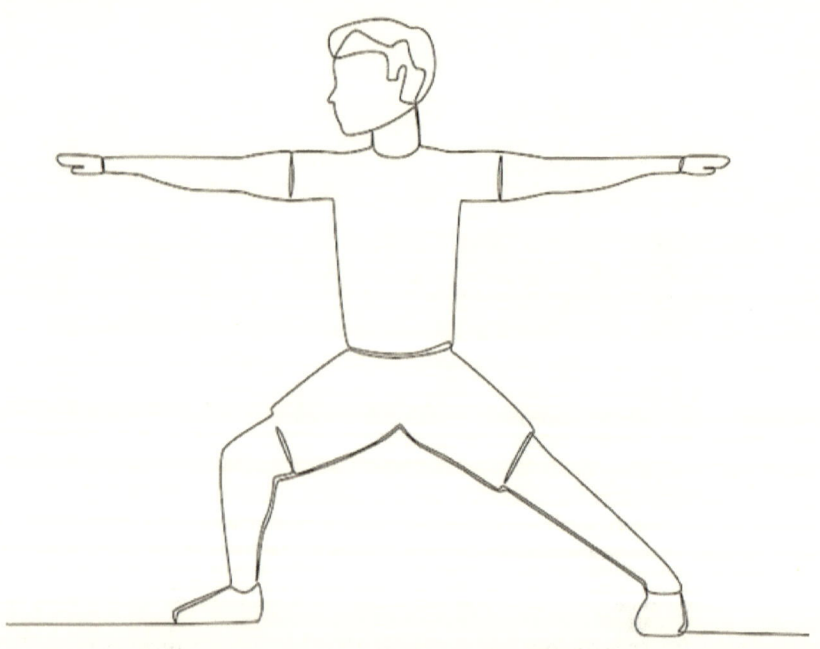

This is a fantastic pose to strengthen your limbs, boost your concentration, improve your balance, enhance blood circulation in the body and helps you become grounded.

To practice it, stand straight on your mat and step your left foot on the back of the mat. Your toes should point at a 45-degree angle in the front. Bend the right knee to keep your thigh parallel to the ground and open the hips on the mat's left side. Your torso should face the left. Extend the right arm towards the mat and the left arm should face the back. Keep them parallel to the ground and reach out through your fingers.

Color Therapy to Balance Your Vata

Colors have an energy of their own, which has different effects on our body, mind and spirit. There are certain colors that beautifully match the energy of the vata dosha and can help balance it if used the right way. Here are some color based remedies you should try to harmonize your unbalanced vata:

Use Blue in Your Everyday Life

The color blue promotes spirituality, independent thinking and imagination. It also reduces fever, keeps you calm and promotes better sleep, which makes it a great color for your vata. Use blue colored objects in your everyday life to benefit from its positivity. for instance, wear at least one blue colored item daily, eat in a blue plate to improve your health problems, use a blue pen to write to promote imaginative thinking and imagine absorbing blue colored light inside you with your eyes closed for 10 minutes once or twice a day.

Green to Your Rescue

The green color has a very soothing effect on your mind, aids metabolism, helps stabilize your body weight and mitigates headaches and fever, which makes it another great color to restore equilibrium to your vata.

Spend time out in a garden or in the forest if possible to absorb the energy of green plants and trees. Moreover, keep a lush plant in your bedroom and workspace to be calm at all times. You can also wear green clothes and keep a few green colored items in your environment.

Purple Heals Pain

Purple reduces stiffness in joints, helps cure angina and increases your self-confidence. When you suffer from joint pains or feel unconfident, use this color to feel better. Keep a purple colored bulb in your room and sit under its light for 30 minutes daily. Also, close your eyes and imagine soft, purple light entering your body and slowly filling your entire system with its warmth and beauty. Imagine the light getting stronger and brighter, and slowly moving out of your body. This calms your vata dosha and helps improve your spirituality, health and overall wellbeing. Do this for 15 minutes daily to benefit from it.

Meditate to Calm Your Mind

Meditation is by far one of the finest and most effective techniques to induce a state of mindfulness so you live in the moment happily and nonjudgmentally, and slowly gain the awareness to make better health, nutrition, fitness, relationship, career and other personal choices for yourself.

Many of us live in a state of forgetfulness which is characterized by living in the past or future, worrying about things that have happened or may happen, letting moments of the present slip by, jumping from one task to another, labeling everything as good or bad, holding judgments and grudges and not enjoying any moment as it comes. This is precisely what induces anxiety, tensions, stress, depression, suicidal thoughts and steers you towards self-harming behaviors, mental disorders and health problems. If only you focus more on living in the moment, life would become fairly simple, easy and beautiful for you.

When you focus on a moment as it comes, do not label your emotions, perceive things for what they are and let go of any pain, grudge and ill sentiment when the moment passes, you do not hold on to any agony or bad memories and just focus on making the best use of every moment. This does wonders to all the 3 doshas and helps you live a harmonious life.

Here is a simple meditative practice for you which if you practice daily can easily promote a state of equilibrium in your mind, body and spirit.

- Sit in a quiet, relaxing place in any pose you like with your eyes closed and hands by your side.

- Inhale through your nose and allow the air to stay in your body for a few seconds before exhaling it. Observe how that makes you feel and try to bring every tiny bit of your attention to that very experience. It will be hard at first, but if you focus on the sensations in your body, the way your belly moves up and down, the way the air circulates in your body and how it inflates your lungs, you will be able to concentrate on the overall experience.

- Slowly exhale through your mouth and focus on the experience again. You need to keep doing that for at least 5 minutes. Just concentrate on how you inhale and exhale, and how that makes you feel.

- When your attention breaks, gently bring it back to your breathing and remind yourself of the important task you are doing now. It will take you a few sessions to become completely focused and invested in the practice, but consistency will help you get there.

- After a few days, meditate by breathing naturally for 2 minutes and then deepen your breath by inhaling for 5 seconds at least and exhaling for 7 or more seconds. The longer you exhale and the more forceful the out-breath is, the more toxins are eliminated out of your system and the more energized you feel.

Work on this technique daily and when you end it, return to your routine chores with a commitment to yourself to do everything mindfully. You will feel extremely calm and with time, you will become more mindful in life. Mindfulness only helps you think, feel and become better, which stabilizes all your doshas.

As you work on restoring balance to your vata dosha, pay attention to your pitta as well. The next chapter discusses ayurvedic techniques to balance your pitta dosha.

Chapter 4: Ayurvedic Practices to Balance Your Pitta Dosha

Of the 3 doshas, the pitta dosha is the oiliest, sharpest and hottest. If you feel extremely hot and exhausted, it could be due to an excess of it. Ayurveda emphasizes on routine detoxification to cleanse your body of waste materials and unnecessary elements.

When too many toxins accumulate in your body and they are not eliminated effectively or timely, you experience an imbalance in your pitta dosha. The toxins are made up of remnants of waste materials, heavy metals, drugs, viruses, bacteria, environmental pollutants, food wastage and any chemicals you ingest.

In Ayurveda, these kind of toxic elements are referred to as 'ama', which is a sticky, heavy and undigested residue that weakens your digestion, process and obstructs the formation of healthy tissues.

You are already aware of the manifestations of a weak and unbalanced pitta; now let us discuss some ayurvedic remedies to bring back that balance. Moreover, many of these practices should be carried out in your everyday routine to achieve optimal harmony in your body and life.

Diet to Balance Your Pitta

Your small intestines and stomach are the two common areas where excess ama often accumulates and these are the two areas you need to pay the most attention to in order to restore balance to your pitta. Here are some diet related guidelines you should observe to achieve that:

- Eat more juicy and sweet fruits like plums, peaches and melons; at least one serving of any of these fruits a day preferably in the morning or afternoon.

- Add some astringent and bitter veggies to your diet such as kale, asparagus and collards as bitterness helps get rid of toxins from your pitta. Observe this only if your vata is balanced.

- Spice up your foods with fennel, turmeric, coriander and cumin as they stabilize your digestion process and soothe any sort of inflammation in your gut.

- Make sure to cut back on your intake of fried, oily, salty, fermented, spicy and hot foods as they make your pitta rough and result in inflammation. This means you should not consume any pickles, kimchi, chilies, crackers and similar foods.

- Slowly cut back on your consumption of caffeine and alcohol, and with time eliminate it for good as these substances are hot and sharp and provoke your pitta.

- Stay hydrated throughout the day by drinking at least 2 liters of clean, drinking water preferably cool water along with fresh fruit and vegetable juices.

Ensure that you work on these practices consistently to yield the desired results. Also, remember to keep your dining room or whatever place you eat in clean and de-cluttered at all times. Cleanliness is an important element in Ayurveda, as a clean environment helps you relax and achieve peace of mind.

Herbs to Balance the Pitta

Herbs are another integral part of Ayurveda and are often used in pitta balancing remedies. Here are some herbs that you should incorporate in your life:

- Neem: It is an incredibly powerful herb as it effectively eliminates toxins from your body especially your blood. It detoxifies the liver, improves your skin health and boosts your immunity. You can use neem in several ways to benefit from it. Boil water with 10 leaves of neem in it and add it to your warm water bath. The healing powers of neem will be absorbed in your body and work their magic on you. While neem leaves are extremely bitter, if you can eat a small piece of it once a day, you will do a huge favor to your body, as it will clear out all the toxins from it and balance your pitta. You can also use neem soaps and shampoos while showering.

- Amalaki: Another helpful herb that cleanses excess ama and supports a healthy digestive process. It also regulates your bowel function and boosts your immunity. Also known as Indian gooseberry, this herb is easily found in its powdered form, which you can add to lemonade or other beverages to enjoy its benefits. You can also add 2 pieces of amalaki along with 5 leaves of kale or spinach and one large apple to prepare a delicious green smoothie full of antioxidants.

Lifestyle Tips to Harmonize Your Pitta

Your lifestyle too plays a huge role in the state of your pitta. The pitta dosha is naturally hot, intense, sharp, acidic and pungent so when it is unbalanced, these characteristics intensify. To restore balance, you need to neutralize its intensity by helping it stay calm, cool and soft. Here are some lifestyle guidelines which if you observe can harmonize the fiery nature of pitta:

- Take cool showers whenever you can and when you feel exhausted. If you are near a river, lake or ocean, visit it as much as you can at least once in 2 weeks to absorb the natural coolness of the river/ocean and calm your pitta.

- Go to bed early to give your pitta enough rest and to absorb the calming energy of the night. The moon has a soft, soothing energy while the sun is invigorating and uplifting. To enjoy both these energies, you need to rest at night and work in the daytime; therefore, make sure that you sleep by 10 or 11pm maximum so that you can wake up around dawn or a little later than that and absorb the power of sunlight. Also, this slowly regulates your circadian rhythm and balances your pitta.

- Massage your body especially abdomen area with coconut or sunflower oil to balance your pitta.

- Do not work for long hours consecutively; instead space out your tasks with short breaks in between. If you work for an hour or two, take a 20 to 30 minute break before moving to the second part of the task or a new task. Your pitta heats up with prolonged activity which then results in frustration, anger and health issues. To avoid that, give your body sufficient rest throughout the day.

- Toxic people harm your pitta just as much as the toxic food does. Therefore, to restore balance to it, distance yourself from negative influences. This includes all those who demotivate you, pull you back and remind you of your failures. Replace such influences with supportive, positive and sweet people who guide, encourage and support you.

- Wear light and cool colored clothes such as shades of green, purple, yellow, white, gray and even pale yellow as these colors soothe your pitta.

- Avoid going out in the sun especially when the UV rays are at their peak, which is around 11am to 4pm mostly as this enrages your pitta and exacerbates your emotional and health issues.

- Plan your work out during the cool hours of the day preferably early morning or late evening. Exercising in the noon or afternoon tends to exhaust your pitta and aggravate your health conditions.

- When the moon is full, spend at least an hour under its light in an open area. Moon bathing does wonders to your entire body especially your stomach and brain, and harmonizes your pitta. This is a practice that you should do at least once a week to absorb the soft, soothing and positive energy of the moon to help your body function optimally.

In addition to these practices, try the following yoga poses to bring your pitta back to the equilibrium state.

Yoga Poses to Calm Down Your Aggravated Pitta

Yoga as you already know has healing and restorative properties and helps your body heal, invigorate and become more flexible. Here are some yoga poses that help you achieve overall balance in the body and improve your emotional and physical health while improving the state of your pitta dosha simultaneously:

Standing Forward Fold

This is a great pose to relieve insomnia, mitigate stress, massage your abdomen, improve digestion and improve your overall fitness and stamina.

To practice it, stand straight with your arms reaching outwards. Slowly bend forward towards your legs and bring your fingers in line with your toes. Plant your palms on the mat/ ground if possible and slowly bend your knees a little without locking them. Draw up your quadriceps muscles and bring your weight slightly forward to your heels. Allow your head to hang over your legs and maintain this pose for 10 to 60 seconds. Take a 20-second break and do it again.

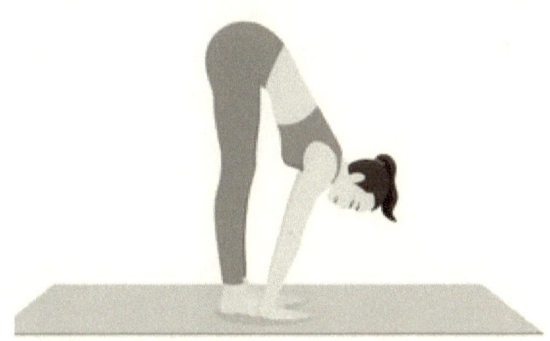

Child's Pose

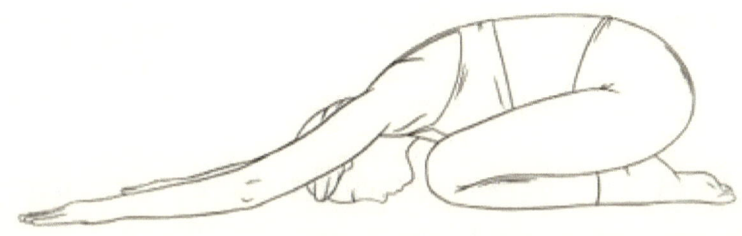

This is another effective and easy to do pose especially for beginners, which massages your internal organs, improves blood circulation, increases awareness and helps you ground. It also helps to relieve stress, anxiety and depression.

To practice it, kneel on the floor and then come in a sitting position with your legs behind you. Gently spread your arms forward on the mat and plant your forehead on the mat. Maintain this pose for 1 to 5 minutes and allow calmness to circulate in your body.

In addition, the poses discussed in the previous chapter help in balancing your pitta too. It is recommended to create a yoga routine using all the poses discussed so far and those that will be discussed in the next chapter and practice them daily to achieve good health, emotional wellbeing and mental contentment.

Now let us move to the next chapter to learn ways to improve the functioning of your kapha dosha.

Chapter 5: Ayurvedic Practices to Balance Your Kapha Dosha

Maintaining a balanced kapha is integral to ensuring that your body functions optimally. Here are some ayurvedic practices that achieve that goal and will ensure that you live a harmonious life:

Create a Balanced, Manageable Routine

Ayurveda emphasizes on balance because that is how you achieve harmony in life. This is especially important for a happy kapha dosha. For that, play your part in creating a manageable routine. Always take up as many tasks as you can handle easily and do not overwhelm yourself by filling your plate with more than your power and ability.

Also, pay attention to your emotions and feelings when you take up a task and if something stresses you out, and you can avoid that task, get rid of it. This helps you become involved in activities you enjoy; thus, improving your emotional wellbeing as well as kapha dosha.

Establish a Morning Routine

Having a healthy morning routine is crucial to becoming a vehement ayurvedic practitioner and to balance your kapha. A morning routine refers to doing certain activities in the morning hours to achieve desired outcomes. Here is a traditional ayurvedic morning routine that you can follow or use to come up with your own to harmonize your imbalanced kapha:

- Wake up at dawn: The ideal time to wake up in Ayurveda is between 3am to 6am, just a little before dawn or right at dawn. This is the time when the atmosphere around you is saturated with energy that clarifies your mind, cleanses your body and helps you become light, energetic and positive. To wake up during this time, sleep around 10pm or maximum 11pm.

- Drink Water Before Emptying Your Bladder: Right when you wake up, drink 2 glasses of clean water and then urinate. It is important to empty your bladder early in the morning to eliminate toxins from it. It is recommended to drink a glass of lukewarm water when you wake up to regulate your gut's functioning and to harmonize your kapha.

- Scrape Your Tongue: Using a stainless steel tongue cleaner, scrape your tongue softly, gently and firmly. This greatly improves your oral hygiene. Do it for 30 seconds daily in the morning. This should be followed by brushing your teeth.

- Practice Oil Pulling: Next, drink a glass of lukewarm water and practice oil pulling which strengthens your jaw, gums, teeth and your gut. It also harmonizes your kapha dosha. To do it, take mustard oil and gargle using it. Spit it out after holding it in your mouth for at least one minute.

- Meditate: Splash cold water on your eyes to awaken your senses, cool your mind and eyes and invigorate your system. Also, this improves your kapha dosha's energy. Next, practice simple breathing meditation for 2 minutes followed by gently chanting any mantra you like. A mantra is a word or a phrase that you chant repeatedly to achieve desired results. You could say 'om', 'peace', 'happiness' or any other thing you would like to manifest in your life. Practice it for 5 to 10 minutes to relax yourself and prepare your body and mind for the tasks lined for the day.

After exercising these practices, try the following yoga poses.

Yoga Poses to Balance Your Kapha

In addition to the yoga poses taught previously, here are 2 more that both do wonders to your flexibility, stamina, strength, balance, focus, cognition, digestion, metabolism and improve your kapha dosha.

Chair Pose

To practice it, stand straight with feet at hip distance apart and then gently move down and slightly backwards as if you are sitting on a chair. Your legs need to be bent and your arms can be extended upwards or placed on your sides. Plant your heels firmly on the ground and your weight should be on your thighs. Practice this pose for 10 to 60 seconds for 3 to 5 times.

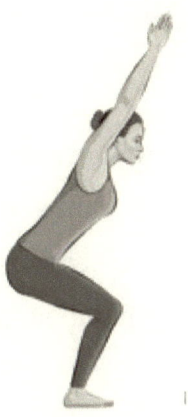

Plank Pose

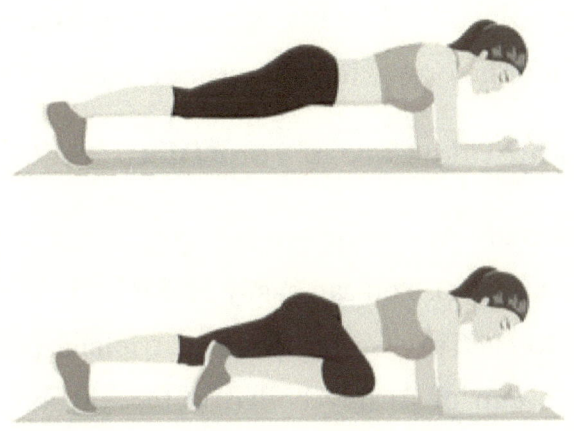

Cartwheel both your hands down on a mat and gently step both the feet backwards. Extend your hips forward until your shoulders move over your wrist. Your body should be in one straight line extending from your head to the heels and your weight should be on your hands.

Do not slouch or let your buttocks drop downwards. Your shoulders must be away from the ears and palms planted firmly on the ground. Maintain this pose for 10 seconds up to 5 minutes or more depending on your strength and stamina.

Oil Massage

Take sesame seed oil and use it to massage your entire body including your ears and toes for 30 minutes at least. It is advisable to warm the oil before massaging it and to practice this remedy an hour before taking a shower or bath.

Use Triphala and Take Care of Your Diet

Tiphala is a customary Ayurvedic formula containing 3 fruits that balance the 3 doshas. You can easily find it in the market and on herbal stores. Take ½ teaspoon of triphala powder and steep it in a cup of freshly boiled water for about 10 minutes. Let it cool and drink it about 30 minutes prior to your bedtime. This energizes your body, soothes your nerves and restores balance to it.

In addition, you should consume low fat milk, reduce your intake of nuts, add honey to milk before consuming it, eat whole wheat grains and fruits such as apples and pears on a regular basis. Nut consumption should be reduced until you restore balance to your kapha. Once it is stabilized, eat nuts but in moderation.

Establish a Healthy Bedtime Routine

You must go to bed early, but it should be at least 3 hours after your last meal so if you wish to sleep at 10pm, you must have dinner by 7 pm and not later. Also, try not to sleep for long hours. On average, adults need 7 to 9 hours of sleep; therefore, try to sleep for 7 to 8 hours at the most, since in Ayurveda, too much sleep creates lethargy, which then creates imbalance in the kapha dosha primarily.

If you stick to these guidelines for good, you will only improve your health and quality of life.

Conclusion

We have come to the end of the book. Thank you for reading and congratulations for reading until the end.

I hope this book serves to be your guide in bringing Ayurveda into your life.